CBD Oil And Hemp Oil:

Using CBD Oil, Hemp Oil, Medical Marijuana And Cannabinoids for General Health Benefits, A Step by Step Guide

Allan McCampbell

Legal & Disclaimer

The information contained in this book is not designed to replace or take the place of any form of medicine or professional medical advice. The information in this book has been provided for educational and entertainment purposes only. The information contained in this book has been compiled from sources deemed reliable, and it is accurate to the best of the Author's knowledge; however, the Author cannot guarantee its accuracy and validity and cannot be held liable for any errors or omissions. Changes are periodically made to this book. You must consult your doctor or get professional medical advice before using any of the suggested remedies, techniques, or information in this book.

Upon using the information contained in this book, you agree to hold harmless the Author from and against any damages, costs, and expenses, including any legal fees potentially resulting from the application of any of the information provided by this guide. This disclaimer applies to any damages or injury caused by the use and application, whether directly or indirectly, of any advice or information presented, whether for breach of contract, tort, negligence, personal injury, criminal intent, or under any other cause of action.

You agree to accept all risks of using the information presented inside this book. You need to consult a professional medical practitioner in order to ensure you are both able and healthy enough to participate in this program.

Table of Contents

Introduction

In the past decade, medical marijuana and cannabis products have been in the limelight a lot. Even people who would never consider taking "drugs" have been interested in the effects of the cannabis plant. I am one of them.

In school, I was a "straight-A student". While my peers drank and smoked who know what, I never even smoked a cigarette. I knew who I could get weed from, and I knew where I could smoke without getting caught. But I didn't smoke. Simply because I knew it was illegal - that was my reason. I had the "drug talk" with my parents, who gave me all the more reason not to get sucked into it. I never considered myself to be "at risk" because I couldn't imagine ever consuming drugs.

I think this is a mentality most people share. They don't want to do drugs and they certainly don't want to do any illegal drugs, which is why anything connected to cannabis is still seen as forbidden.

Over the past few years, CBD has become quite popular - maybe because it doesn't make you high like marijuana does, and because it's still in a legal grey area. I want to emphasize that CBD falls under the Schedule I Classification, which means that it's technically illegal unless you have medical requirements.
Since countless people starting giving CBD a try after having been failed by conventional treatment, many more became willing to give it a try despite its questionable legality. I was one of those people.
I suffer from nerve pain and nerve damage. Painkillers do not work on me, and when the nerve is triggered it feels like being stabbed in the back by a bolt of lightning that slowly works its way down to my feet. It's like having a current drain your insides until there's nothing you can do but cry out in pain and try not to make it any worse.
There are days I can't walk.
My doctors put me on antidepressants, but they only messed up my brain. Epilepsy medication gives me severe anxiety, and antispasmodics don't help either because my problem isn't a muscular one.

CBD and cannabis products gave me an alternative that so far hasn't only kept the lightning bolts at bay but also improved my mood. They did what Western medicine couldn't, and I don't even feel like I'm taking drugs because I'm not getting high. My mind is just a lot less messed up now.

All this is why I want more people to know about CBD and cannabis products. Not for the hype or the infamous curative effects but so that people have a viable alternative to traditional medicine.

I'm not a doctor, but I've quickly become a believer and an advocate because of what it's done for me. Cannabis products have basically given me my life back, and I want to share what convinced me, a true skeptic, to give them a try.

-Allan

Thank you so much for your support through buying and reading this book, it means the world to me!

If you never want to miss out on one of my future books, consider signing up for my newsletter here

http://bit.ly/allannewsletter

and checking out my author's page here

http://amzn.to/allanmccampbell

Chapter 1 – How to Use This Book

Most readers who are looking to use CBD and medical marijuana find that the information is pretty lacking. There's tons of information on scientific studies on the internet but hardly any of it goes into terminology, abbreviations or dosage guidelines. For those that don't live in a place where these products have been legalized or at least decriminalized, acquiring the "goods" can be tricky without a prescription or a how-to guide.

The information in this book can seem daunting at first, but it's equally helpful at the very least.

1. If you're looking to find out which medical conditions can be treated with CBD oil, read Chapters 5-7. Moreover, Chapter 7 contains information on CBD dosing for pets, including some recipes. You should also check out Chapter 4 to learn about delivery methods.

2. If you're interested in understanding the difference between psychoactive and non-

psychoactive cannabis as well as the spectrum between them, Chapter 3 should be particularly useful for you. Chapter 2 will familiarize you with the ins and outs of medical marijuana.

That being said, the best thing for you is to determine what you want and what your limits are. If there are any terms you're unsure of, refer back to the terminology section and bookmark any portions you might need to look at more closely.

This book is by no means without flaws, but I've tried to include as much information as possible to help you get started. The way CBD works has got everything to do with the receptors in your body. These differ from person to person, which is why it's hard to say how similar your experience will be to mine.

Common Terminology

At this point, you've probably seen several words that you don't understand. I'll try and explain them as we go along, but here's a short definition guide that should help you get a general understanding.

- **Cannabis** - another word for marijuana or hemp. It refers to the plant itself but can also denote the dried leaves.

- **Strain** - a variety of plant. Think of it as the botanical equivalent of a dog breed. The strain denotes the type of plant and what it is best used for.

- **Cannabinoid** - a chemical extracted from the cannabis plant. Cannabinoids, by nature, are not psychoactive.

- **Hemp** - the strain of cannabis plant most commonly used for ropes, bird seeds, and CBD production. It is low in THC but high in Cannabinoids.

- **THC** - delta-9-tetrahydrocannabinol. This is the compound found in cannabis plants that causes the "high" and also the "active ingredient" in medical marijuana. THC is the psychoactive part of the marijuana plant.

- **Endocannabinoid** - a cannabinoid produced by the human body.

- **CBD** - cannabidiol, a compound rich in cannabinoids. It is usually refined as an oil or extract.

- **Marijuana** - a term applied to both the cannabis plant as a whole and the dried leaves/buds that are harvested to make medical marijuana.

Legal Considerations

Despite what people may tell you, CBD is not legal. Marijuana has been legalized in several parts of the US (e.g. Colorado, Washington DC, and California) on a state level, but it remains a Schedule 1 drug federally. It is only legal to use CBD products if you have a certified prescription for them.

I don't think it will be long before other parts of the world follow suit. Due to the medical benefits of marijuana, many countries already have relaxed regulations, and even though these don't give you a free pass, it's the first step to global legalization.

Chapter 2 - Marijuana as Medicine

Marijuana was one of the first plants to be used medicinally, with traces of seed and plant debris being found in prehistoric settlements. The unique nature of this plant means that Cannabidiol is actually the largest Phytocannabinoid in existence, and while there are over 100 different ones, it is this one that has the most medical benefits. Hemp, on the other hand, was one of the world's first cultivated crops.

While some people think that medical cannabis is new, the practice of using herbs and plants against ailments dates back to prehistoric times. There's no reason why cannabis couldn't have been used back then, and while science has always been skeptical of herbal cures, the success of drugs like willow bark aspirin shows that herbalists aren't just wannabe healers.

Marijuana History

Back in 2009, the justice department made history by saying they would no longer pursue medical users of marijuana who complied with state drug laws. While the number of states that allow marijuana for medical purposes is growing steadily, this landmark decision meant that there was protection from federal level prosecution. The historical use of marijuana as a medicine dates as far back as 2737 BC - to China where marijuana was used to treat malaria, gout, and rheumatism. Emperor Shen Neng used cannabis tea to treat a variety of conditions. It then spread through Asia and Africa and also gained some religious following. Physicians began to prescribe it to ease everything from childbirth to memory loss. However, even then there were warnings about overuse.

Ancient Egyptian texts document cannabis as treatment for tumors. It was also frequently used in ancient Greece, the Roman Empire and various other ancient civilizations. Due to their skepticism and concern over the psychoactive aspect, the Greeks were one of the last to embrace cannabis treatments. Ironically, they were also one of the first modern countries to ban it.

By the 18th century, it was pretty common for medical journals to feature information on hemp and cannabis as cures. Dr. William O'Shaughnessy first brought their use to England and America as a ship's physician of the British East India Company, and his studies showed good effects on inflammations and rheumatism. The issue was that during the 19th century, the morphine epidemic led the American government to crackdown on opioids. At the time, marijuana was safe, but it was a shift in the regulation of anything "medical".

The Harrison Act of 1914 criminalized the use of marijuana by introducing a tax so high that it made it unattainable for most, and not paying the tax was a big crime. By 1937, 23 states had decided to make marijuana illegal because chasing tax dodgers took too much time. The Marihuana [sic] Tax Act made non-medical use illegal, exempting only hempseeds when used as birdseeds, and this still applies today. Even today, the state department insists on this antiquated spelling for some reason.

The laws were less strict in the 1970s, but Reagan Era politics cracked down on many liberal leanings. It wasn't until 1996, when California first legalized medical marijuana, that things once again began to relax.

Over the last two decades, researchers have extensively studied cannabis and CBD as a separate cannabinoid for medical use without the psychoactive effects of CBD. In the last 10 years, these studies have had promising results despite marijuana remaining a Schedule 1 drug. The issue is that much of the highest grade CBD is made from medical grade cannabis, something only available in "legal" states. While there's less danger from interfering chemical agents than in other illegal drugs, many dubious supplies aren't as refined or as pure, meaning the actual cannabidiol content might not be high enough to get the expected results.

As the use of medical marijuana is not currently allowed on a particularly large scale, many barriers exist for researchers and distributors. FDIC banks, for example, cannot fund or give loans to individuals involved with CBD. Because of this "cash only" status, the huge security risk for businesses, the many insurance issues and interstate transport are just some of the reasons research has been stalled.

Despite all this, however, the organization that started the promotion of marijuana as a therapy drug in the 1960s has swelled. Much of the advances that marijuana research has made in the 21st century has to do with compassion. Seeing people suffer when they could be enjoying life makes the public at large sympathetic and more supportive of the work researchers are doing.

While holistic remedies are still handled with much skepticism, many forget that the same remedies were often proven right with research. Aspirin, for example, is nothing more than a refined willow bark, and new research suggests that honey and oregano may be effective against MRSA. The use of marijuana is becoming more mainstream, and it's very likely we will see wider legalization across the globe in the next decade, which would scientifically support claims advocacy movements have been making for the past 50 years.

Legality Medical Marijuana vs CBD

Here's the thing - while medical marijuana is only just becoming legal, CBD is completely legal in the majority of US states. This is because much like the hemp birdseed production, which was exempted in 1937, CBD oil has no psychoactive effects. You cannot "get high" on CBD oil. It is still an international grey area. In December of 2016, however, the DEA ruled that CBD, being an "extract", is still considered a Schedule 1 drug and therefore subject to tracking.

Even though you can buy CBD oil online from reputable companies (even Amazon), it is technically still not a legal substance.

Most companies get around this by using the hemp plant for CBD oil. While essentially the same plant, hemp and marijuana have different strains and entirely different uses because of their diverging chemical structure. You cannot get "high" from a hemp plant because the percentage of THC, the chemical used to make you high, is so low (0.3%) that it's basically considered legal.

The legal situation is actually kind of a mess because it regulates something called cannabidiol, a cannabinoid, and the problem is that cannabinoids come in many forms, including those in your own body. How can something you yourself produce naturally be an illegal substance? There is no legitimate way to ban cannabinoids, which is why CBD neither fits the medical marijuana nor the controlled substance laws.

The DEA reasons that CBD oil has no other cannabinoids is it legal, something that is entirely impossible even for the purest extraction process. It is still possible to be prosecuted just for having the oil regardless of whether it is derived from a marijuana plant or a hemp plant.

There are now 16 states that have specific CBD laws. They apply to patients using non-psychoactive CBD, but obtaining it is still not entirely legal.

If you consider using CBD, I want you to be certain that this is something you really want and can handle. After all, even though many do use it daily without government interference, it is still considered a Schedule I drug. This means that, in the eyes of the law, possession is no different from regular marijuana.

Ethnobiology of CBD Cannabis Plants

With plants used to recreationally "get high", it's understandable that skeptics worry that legalization is nothing more than an effort to legalize moral deficiency. Intuitively, most users know whether cannabis affects them positively or negatively, but many of the staunchest opponents either see no benefits for themselves or simply do not understand the motivation behind legalization.

Patients like the PTSD-afflicted, elderlies who want arthritis relief, cancer sufferers, or a baby with seizures are not trying to "get high", which is why CBD is much more appealing to them. After all, a single CBD dose can do more for them than years of traditional treatment options.

Clinicians and other medical professionals that see the struggles people on conventional meds go through first-hand are often the first to realize that the cultural attitude towards CBD is changing. After almost a century of scrutinizing cannabis, compassion and scientific evidence are beginning to win out over greed and prejudice.

States like California are flooding the market with specific strains, but researchers have found that biodiversity of high CBD strains is a better way to go. For modern pharmacopoeia to be effective, it needs to include all strains of the plant, something that researchers are still struggling to get access to. In fact, it may be this narrowing of varieties that is responsible for the lack of a "breakthrough" result.

Cannabis itself is a synergistic poly-pharmaceutical. This means that it's made of many different interacting components, which is especially important for CBD because without the phyto-compound terpenes the side effects of THC become too severe. For the most effective result, all parts of a plant should be used to get the balance right.

Versions of CBD Medications

Cannabis medication comes in a variety of different forms, depending on what the treatment needs are.

The most common CBD drug is Sativex (nabiximols), which has been approved in 24 countries with a 1:1 ratio of CBD to THC. It is usually the first cannabis prescription issued to cancer patients and administered as a sublingual spray.

Epidiolex (cannabidiol) is used for epilepsy treatment. Studies have shown that this is the most effective anticonvulsant of plant-based CBD medications.

Almost all other varieties of cannabis medication are THC-based.

Synthetic cannabinoids are man-made and can be consumed in as many forms as traditional CBD (inhaled, sprayed, etc.). These are called cannabinoids because they are chemically similar and activate the same receptors as naturally derived CBD. They are marketed as a "safe" and "legal" form because they are not actually derived from cannabis. However, since they are technically still classified as Schedule 1, they are neither safe nor legal. The effects can be unpredictable and are often stronger because they are not naturally derived and less regulated. Synthetic manufacturers usually license synthetic cannabinoids as incense to get around the procedural licensing requirements.

Synthetic CBD is commonly used as an additive in prescription meds, but on its own it has very little medical benefits.

Matching Strains to Conditions

There are over 1,000 different strains of cannabis. The name of a strain is often the only thing a patient is given when deciding what type of product to use, but the number of choices seems daunting regardless. What you need to know about strains is that they all have different effects. The most important thing to consider is the ratio between CBD and THC as well as the terpene content.

The three main strains you'll encounter are sativa, indica, ruderalis and their hybrids. One strain may work better for you than others, and because not all plants within a strain have the same genetic traits it's not quite possible to say which one would work best.

Many varieties are dependent on the nutrients and growing techniques used to cultivate that particular variety. Plants are cloned repeatedly until there is enough for a crop. Most CBD plants are only available as a cloned variety, which means getting the same effects from homegrown plants as from artificial products is practically impossible.

The seeds themselves can also differ because some will be female with a different CBD:THC ratio. Cloning helps prevent differences but because of specific growing methods, it can still happen.
Cannabis is the genus of a plant, while the strain determines the subspecies.

Sativa

Sativa originated in Mexico and Southeast Asia. It has narrow leaves with thin branches that are more widespread than Indica or Ruderalis. These are smaller plants with few flowers. The effects of sativa are usually more cerebral and less sedative because it has a higher level of the enzyme needed to convert CBG into CBD. It has a greater stimulant and energizing effect that increases focus and creativity. It does make you more susceptible to paranoia, increased anxiety, hyperactivity, and an increased heart rate though.

Indica

Indica strains come from the Kush region in the Middle East (Morocco, Turkey, Afghanistan, India etc.). They grow better in cooler climates and at high altitudes. The plant has broad leaves and is the bushiest of the strains. It provides a more relaxing experience and less energizing effects. It relieves muscle pain, promotes sleep, relieves pain and spasms, reduces seizures, and reduces stress. However, it might make you feel more tired, sluggish and unmotivated. Overeating is a side effect as well. The Indica strain is the classic "stoner" variety.

Ruderalis

This is the last of the subspecies and the most varied. Leaf size varies between strains and is sometimes closer to Indica and at other times closer to Sativa. It is short like an Indica plant and less cultivated, which often gives it the name of "wild" cannabis. It was identified in Russia in 1924 and grows in the wilderness of southern Siberia, mostly on rough ground. It is also where the term "ditch weed" comes from. It has very low levels of THC and high levels of cannabinol, which makes it more attractive for CBD use.

Hybrids

Hybrid strains are generally created specifically for either THC or CBD properties. The plants may also be coded based on the precursor acids present in the raw plant.
No matter which strain CBD is extracted from, it is always the same molecule. The only difference is the amount harvested per plant, something that is irrelevant unless you are planning on growing and extracting your own product. CBD can be extracted from industrial hemp because of the low THC content, but the best kinds are from CBD-rich strains instead. As with many products, China is a big producer of cheap industrial hemp, which leads to plenty of substandard CBD products becoming available cheaply. The FDA and DEA cautions specifically against using these because they may contain dangerous additives and impurities, and many of the claims about them are unsubstantiated.

The "gold standard" for CBD strains is AC/DC. It is a type of Cannatonic hybrid that has a ratio of 22:1, which is why it is the first strain that patients are advised to try if interested in this alternative approach. Not only is it the most effective, but it also has very little THC in it. It has a well-rounded profile and was propagated in 2011 by Dr. William Courtney from Spanish Cannatonic seeds that were then cloned. The term AC/DC stands for Alternative Cannabinoid/Dietary Cannabis because of the high raw CBD content. It is a 50/50 hybrid between an Indica and a Sativa strain.

Cannatonic was the first CBD-rich strain to prompt the interest in CBD products. It is a valuable, widely available strain and frequently featured in "success stories".

Chapter 3 – The Biology of Cannabis

The effect cannabis has on the body depends on how the plant is constructed. In the 1970s, neurotransmitter chemicals, the chemical messengers used by the body and brain to communicate, were discovered. These chemicals regulate and organize every major system within the body, and the messages between neurons are responsible for transmitting everything from brain to body.

The Endocannabinoid System

For the neurotransmitter to work there have to be neuroreceptors. These protein molecules are found within cell membranes that allow communication to pass between one cell wall and the next. Researchers found receptor sites in the brain that were activated by opioids, and it wasn't long before it was discovered that the same receptors react to cannabis.

The problem was that the political agenda of the time focused on funding studies to link the two and prove detrimental effects rather than potential benefits.

The latest research into how cannabis affects the body has found an entire endocannabinoid system dedicated specifically to the body's natural version of the chemicals found in cannabis. This system is responsible for two things – to help heal the body in case of injury and to modulate pleasure for complete wellbeing. It's one of the most complex systems, and yet our understanding of it is only basic. Only 13% of medical schools teach the endocannabinoid system, so it's understandable that many in the field of medicine are still skeptical about it.

There are currently several recognized components of the endocannabinoid system – two types of CB receptors, two types of signaling molecules, and five different enzymes. In addition to these, the system also works in tandem with other systems within the body to accomplish its duty. The unique thing about these components is that the receptors are the only part that is permanently there; the rest is simply kept so that the body can use it if needed.

Active Compounds

Everyone has head of THC and CBD, but there are actually a huge number of different chemicals within the cannabis plant that have therapeutic uses. Most of these are unique to the cannabis plant. THC is a phytocannabinoid, whereas CBD is an endocannabinoid. They're chemically different but still exhibit some similarities. Phytocannabinoids work all over the body and are present at all times in our natural structure. Part of the reason it's impossible to overdose on phytocannabinoids is that the body has its own system to regulate them. Drugs and prescriptions that limit endocannabinoid receptors are known to cause brain damage, psychosis, and even death.

One of the first endocannabinoids discovered and classified was Cannabidiol or CBD. Researchers were actually looking for psychoactive THC. They were surprised to find that CBD didn't interact with either CB receptor that they had identified and found it worked independently by blocking the FAAH enzyme used in the endocannabinoid system to regulate anandamide. Currently 11 different phytochemicals have been identified and found to have corresponding effects within the body:

- 9-THC – analgesic, anti-inflammatory, anti-oxidant, anti-epileptic, euphoriant, neuroprotective, anti-emetic, analgesic, anxiolytic
- CBD – anti-cancer, anti-emetic, antipsoriatic, anti-diarrheal, analgesic, anti-inflammatory, antibacterial, anti-diabetic, anxiolytic, antispasmodic, vasorelaxant, anti-psychotic, anti-epileptic, neuroprotective
- 9-THCV – appetite suppressant, anti-epileptic, anti-lipidemia, anti-diabetic, bone stimulant
- CBG – antibacterial, anti-proliferative
- CBC – analgesic, anti-fungal, anti-inflammatory, anti-microbial
- CBDA – anti-cancer, anti-emetic, anti-inflammatory
- 9-THCA – antispasmodic, anti-inflammatory, anti-emetic, euphoric, neuroprotective
- CBDV – bone stimulant

- CBN - analgesic, anti-cancer, anti-inflammatory

The majority of those compounds are not psychoactive or phytocannabinoids but endocannabinoids derived from CBD. While the therapeutic benefits of THC are undeniable, it still has its disadvantages, so it makes sense that CBD is more medically promising. There are 421 different chemical compounds in cannabis and about ¼ of them are phytocannabinoids like THC.

This is one of the reasons many people prefer medical marijuana to CBD products -because it's a combination of these phytocannabinoids and other compounds of the plant for an ideal balance.

One of the reasons that this is a problem for most people interested in CBD is that studies have shown that pure CBD is not as widely effective as whole plant marijuana. In fact, the actual treatment of pain and inflammation is only narrowly effective, while a CBD-enriched plant extract that also contains low levels of the other compounds provides improved anti-inflammatory and pain relief. Essentially, without a bit of THC, CBD is limited in its effectiveness.

The fact that THC works on more non-cannabinoid receptors means that it may be more effective for patients than CBD in some cases.

It probably seems strange to you that I say CBD isn't as effective without THC in a book promoting CBD. It's actually specific to pure medical grade CBD and since our endocannabinoid system is very complex, is it makes sense that the most compatible compound (THC) would have greater effect than CBD, even if the effects are similar.

CBD plays a greater role in connecting the endocannabinoid system and the central nervous system by inhibiting non-cannabinoid receptors and blocking inflammatory processes. CBD is unique in that it converts fats and protects from heart muscle deterioration. The synergy between CBD and THC, however, has shown to be essential in treating certain diseases.

The interesting thing about both compounds is that while both compounds are present in the plant, their quantity increases when heated. This means that a dosing which heats the plant like vaporizing, smoking, or pre-cooking increases the amount of therapeutic chemicals within it. Studies have shown that blood levels are up to 4 times higher compared to raw plant studies even though the psychoactive effects were far lower in raw users.

How the Body Processes Cannabis

You've probably noticed that a lot of what separates marijuana and CBD is all down to science. It really does come down to the molecules inside the plant and the part of the plant itself to determine what makes CBD. THC as such is psychoactive, it will affect your mind in a variety of different ways. It has medical benefits of its own. To understand the difference between the two and the effect of your own cannabinoids, you have to learn how things work within your body.

CB Receptors

Cannabinoids within the oil are treated the exact same by the body as those produced within the body. Your cells can't tell the difference between a cannabinoid produced by a cannabis plant and one produced by your own enzymes. Your body has receptors in it, much like a plug socket, which these cannabinoids attach to so that they can be used. There are two different types of cannabinoid receptors - CB1 and CB2. Depending on where these receptors are located, they have different purposes and designs.

Most CB1 receptors are found in the brain, and the cannabinoids which attach to these are those associated with emotions, appetite, mood, coordination and some pain responses. The shape of the receptor is actually better suited for THC molecules rather than CBD molecules, which is why the CBD does not have such a psychoactive effect. CB2 receptors are found all over the body and are much more common. They are linked to general pain and immune issues.
Within the brain there are 6 parts that have the most CB receptors.

- Basal Ganglia - responsible for movement control
- Cerebellum - responsible for coordination
- Hippocampus - responsible for learning and memory
- Cerebral Cortex - responsible for higher cognitive function
- Intrabulbar Anterior - responsible for linking the two hemispheres
- Nucleus Accumbens - responsible for rewards

While science has figured out that it's the connection of cannabinoids to these receptors that cause certain responses, it's not known why the plant molecules work the same as the body's own.

The body produces cannabinoids to lessen the feeling of pain, boost mood, and lower inflammation. These cannabinoids are a natural response and part of what makes runners feel "high" after exercising.

Studies have shown that not everyone has the same amount or distribution of these CB receptors, which is why some people are more affected by cannabinoids than others. It also explains why some people react so well to marijuana while others experience terrible side effects. It's been shown that those who have a low pain tolerance and those who suffer from chronic pain both have higher numbers of CB receptors, which is why they may find cannabinoid treatments more effective than conventional drugs. It's simply the way their bodies are built.

You can see why this is such a subjective rather than definitive issue. Scientists cannot definitively state that CBD works for pain because on some people it doesn't while on others it will. The effectiveness of CBD is determined on a case by case basis.

Why Cannabinoids Are Not Psychoactive

THC binds to CB1 receptors and, just like cannabinoids mimic those produced in the body, it mimics another chemical so the body processes it as if it was that chemical. THC is molecularly similar to anandamide, a neurotransmitter also called the "bliss molecule". Anandamide is an endocannabinoid that increases pleasure, especially from food, and it is partially what makes up the "runner's high". It has also been linked to memory and pain responses.

Medical marijuana varieties of cannabis plants are bred primarily for their THC levels and not their CBD. While there are some strains which have high CBD levels, there are no medical marijuana strains with no THC, which is why it's easier to use CBD and continue on with life as normal. Medical Marijuana stimulates both CB1 and CB2 receptors, but its primary response is towards CB1, which is why you will always experience an (albeit varied) level of high.

CBD doesn't fit well with these CB1 receptors so the blissful reaction doesn't happen. It's not actively stopping the CB1 receptors but it does antagonize them. When cannabinoids and THC are both present, they cancel each other out and produce a middle ground so you can still get high while ingesting CBD, although you won't get that high. Similarly, the effects of CBD will be minimized by the presence of THC because the CB1 receptors are being repressed. CBD prevents the bad side of THC from becoming too strong, but it limits the high. By taking away the THC entirely, there simply is no high, and by having such a low THC percentage, the effect on the CB1 receptors is simply overwhelmed by the CB2 response instead.

You simply cannot get high from CBD unless it's mixed with THC, which CBD oil is not. In fact, the extraction process usually removes the THC or uses an entirely different part of the plant.

Anatomy of a Cannabis Plant

Cannabis plants are not simple and come in both male and female varieties. They have buds at the top which contain the flowers and produce the branches and leaves. The leaves will eventually grow out of the clump and become the recognizable fan shape. The bud is only found on the female plant, which grows in a tight cluster of buds called a cola. One plant may have many colas on it, but there's usually an atypical "prime" bud at the very top of the plant.

The bud is made up of the flowering parts of the plant (stigma, bract, calyx) and, it is actually where you find the highest concentration of cannabinoids and THC. The stigma are the small, hairy bits sticking out from the bud, and the main part of the calyx is covered in a sticky resin which protects where CBD comes from. This resin covers the delicate trichome where the majority of the plant oils are excreted, including terpenes, CBD and THC.

CBD strains of cannabis are different from THC strains but they're not visibly much different from any other variety. There are in fact, 85+ different varieties or strains of cannabis. Within the bud, the percentage of CBD or THC is what determines whether that strain is better for hemp production or for marijuana. Plants that have over 4% CBD are considered to be high, and usually not suited for marijuana production. Common CBD strains include Charlotte's Web, Cannatonic, and Sour Tsunami among others. There are fewer strains which produce high CBD than those that are high in THC.

Why Hemp Is Not CBD

In theory, since hemp plants are low in THC, there is no reason they should be illegal, but because of the grey area described in chapter 1, it's not that simple. There are two different types of hemp oil - hempseed and hemp extract. Hempseed oil comes from plants that have no THC and almost no CBD at all. In fact, there's usually >0.00000025% cannabidiol in hemp oil, while CBD can be as concentrated as 20%. It's generally used in food production for this reason and perfectly legal. It is high in Omega-3 amino acids, which is why it's good for food production. While there are differences between the seed and extract oils, neither contains enough cannabidiol to be useful.

Hemp oil uses the stalk and seed rather than the bud and is rich in 400 different phytonutrients. Phytonutrients are found in all varieties of fruits and vegetables and are part of what keeps our immune system healthy and protected from free radical damage. It's often used in the same way as coconut oil or vegetable shortening. It's high in GLAs, which is why some people use it for eczema and skin issues.

Unlike both CBD and THC, hemp oil can have some nasty side effects. Hemp oil has been linked to hallucinations, paranoia, and inflammation. The issue is that hemp is also high in Omega-6 fatty acids, and these cause immunosuppression, inflammation, and cardiac issues. They increase the risk of cancer and can cause coagulation issues. Like red palm oil, it can also cause digestive upset and disrupt the cells in the digestive tract. It's prohibited for pregnant women because it can affect them and the baby's development. Despite being marketed as a health product, hemp oil is actually not healthy at all.

Be aware that the two terms are not interchangeable when buying products. Hemp and CBD oils are very different.

Chapter 4 – CBD Oil and Dosing

Most plant extracts are made using one of three common methods. The method of extraction is very important because it will determine the purity of the oil and the chances of contamination. The purer the oil the more concentrated and the less chance of any unwanted side effects from contaminants. Purer oils tend to cost more because the process is more time-consuming and more expensive. All cannabis plants produce some level of CBD, but because it's higher in hemp plants, it's often confused with hemp oil. Remember, the two are NOT the same thing!

Producing CBD Oil

There are three main extraction methods that apply to CBD:

- CO2 Extraction - This is the most scientific, pure, and expensive method. High-pressure CO2 gas is blasted at the plant until it is completely dry. The oil and resin are then collected from the plant. It removes the chlorophyll and has no residue, which is why it's the purest but - because of the equipment and technicality of the method - also the most industrial and impossible to "make at home". Think of this as the "organic, therapeutic grade" of essential oils.

- Oil Extraction - You've probably seen peppers or herbs in oil before for cooking. Placing any plant into oil causes the oils inside the plant to seep into the oil around, flavoring and infusing the carrier oil over time. The whole bud is submerged into a carrier oil until the oil becomes infused. Depending on the carrier oil, there may be additional benefits. There is no residue in this method, provided the carrier oil is pure and the plant has been cleaned of pesticides before submerging. This can be done at home, but the type of plant matters most as THC will also infuse this way.

- Ethanol Extraction - This works much like the oil method but uses a high percentage alcohol volume instead of an oil. The extract is separated later and put into a (usually cheaper) carrier oil. The issue with using grain alcohol is that it leaves a slight residue and denatures the oil slightly so there is a specific taste. It also destroys terpenes and other beneficial natural compounds that usually infuse with the CBD. It's cheap and while it can still be called pure (because nothing other than the chemicals used and the cannabinoids are present), the chemicals remain behind in the finished product. While this can be done at home, it's going to have the same effect as oil infusion and will give you cannabis alcohol rather than CBD because the alcohol extraction process can't be done at home.

Concentrated CBD

CBD concentrates are the most popular form for therapy because they have the highest dose of cannabinoids compared to all other dosing methods. The problem is that they are often confusing because of their variety. Concentrated CBD oil is more concentrated than the plant itself and often referred to by many names like crumble, shatter, wax, RSO, or kief.

Extracting CBD is usually done with one of the three methods above except for RSO. RSO stands for Rick Simpson Oil - it was the first method of extraction to become popular. The first extractions used rather toxic chemicals and solvents like butane and hexane, and while these are supposed to be "removed" by the extraction process, there's only few chemists that have actually done any tests to confirm this. It is similar to Butane Hash Oil or BHO, which is the cheapest and most widely available grey market CBD. It uses butane to extract the oil and is not only highly flammable but can also have a noticeable reside left from the process.

Most CBD wax products are made using BHO, and these are not only the lowest concentrations but also the most dangerous because of the higher chance of contamination. It is not advised to smoke any CBD product that has been extracted using solvent methods.

Kief

This is the most natural CBD concentrate - it is made from the crystals that dry cannabis buds. It is filtered and made into a fine powder.

Hash

Hash is one of the oldest forms of CBD and made using a non-solvent form where the plants are layered, pressed, dried, and the tar scraped off and rolled into balls. It is often a manual process, making it expensive compared to chemically extracted concentrates.

Rosin or Resin

This is often a side product from smoking, and most users will explain about scraping resin from the inside of their apparatus to keep it clean. The heating process is simple and solvent-free and simply heats the trichomes of the plant to increase the potency of the CBD before pressing the oils out.

CO2 Oil

This is an expensive method, but it is the purest as detailed above because it undergoes a secondary process to remove the solvents.

Side Effects of CBD

Since CBD is not psychoactive, most of the side effects are quite minimal. Most people feel no negative effects at all. The most common side effects of CBD are dry mouth and low blood pressure. Low blood pressure, in turn, can show up as dizziness, nausea, drowsiness, and lightheadedness. Because of the marked effect on blood pressure, CBD is quite dangerous for patients who have cardiac issues or rely on anticoagulants. Patients on these are told not to eat citrus and especially grapefruit because they contain the same compounds. It inhibits hepatic drugs and decreases the proteins needed for the liver to metabolize medications in general. If you're also using conventional medication, it's important to consult with your doctor before mixing the two.

As CBD may cause drowsiness, it's important to be careful when you start using it and avoid driving or operating machinery that could be dangerous. While CBD isn't psychoactive and will not show up on a drug test, it is still mood-altering. There's a low chance of being allergic to CBD itself, but most people who suffer side effects get them from cheap oils and contaminants rather than the CBD itself.
Avoiding cheap oil and those which aren't pure can help negate the chances of any reactions, but don't simply buy an expensive oil because you think it's purer - look at the extraction methods above and research the company first.

Dosing with Cannabis

CBD medication is much easier to take than one high in THC because it's not psychoactive. The effects are not mind altering so it's possible to feel calmer and more relaxed. However, individuals who are sensitive to THC may still have a small but similar reaction to normal users when taking CBD. If you're not used to cannabis products, it's essential not to use a car or machine until you know how your body will react. The effects of the products often have to do with the strain and biochemistry of the plant.

To find the correct dosing, you should consider the condition or problem you are trying to treat, the intensity of the problem, how you respond to CBD, your weight, age and how sensitive you are to medications and chemicals as well as whether your body adapts easily.
While CBD is generally safe, being cautious and building up dosage using a method called "titration" to slowly adjust is considered the most effective. Adjusting slowly upwards and with caution means you are less likely to experience a significantly negative effect from a bad reaction.
The three dose ranges are micro, standard and macro.

Micro Dose

A micro dose is the lowest available dose for CBD medications. It has a range of 05.5-20mg per dose per day. It is usually used for PTSD, stress, nausea, headaches, sleep disorders and metabolic problems.

Standard Dose

The standard dose falls into the middle range, which is usually between 10mg to 100mg per dose a day. It sometimes overlaps with the lowest micro dose because many people who take a micro dose actually end up with a standard dose when they take multiple doses a day without realizing it. Standard doses are used for autoimmune disorders, anxiety, arthritis, fibromyalgia, MS, IBS, autism, pain, Lyme disease, and some mental health issues.

Macro Dose

This is the strongest CBD dose, and it's usually between 50mg to 800mg per dose per day. This is usually used for treating cancer and life-threatening condition like epilepsy and seizures. It is considered a therapeutic dose rather than an herbal one.

Reaching the macro dose level usually means a period of 4-6 weeks of acclimatization with a dosing increase every 3-4 days so that the body can tolerate it without any negative side effects.

Another way to take the macro dose if you are combining THC and CBD is to take the CBD during the day and the THC at night to negate the sedative effect.

To determine your best dose, choose which of these best fits your purpose for CBD, then go by weight to find the ideal dose. For instance, if you have a 1:1 ratio with 20mg, then only 10mg of that will be CBD. How you divide that dose is up to you - determine your comfort level and continue for 2-4 days to determine how it works for you. If you experience any negative effects, you should halve your next dose. If you are using titration, you can increase your dose every 2-3 days or by 20% and then observe your reactions. Your target dose should be below the one that gives you a negative reaction but above the one before that.

The more you weigh, the higher your dose of CBD will be. There is no "one size" dosing method because everyone has different numbers of receptors, and different dosing methods will change the effectiveness of the CBD absorption.

Tolerance

Over time, many people develop a tolerance for cannabis. How quickly your body does this often depends on your genetic makeup and the strength of the product you are using. Many find they have to slowly raise their dose over time to reach the same effectiveness, which is why cannabis is often considered addictive. The higher the dose and the more frequently you use it, the quicker the CB1 receptors become desensitized.

To get around this, the best thing is to take a break of 3-4 days every few months. Since your fat cells have stored cannabinoids, you shouldn't experience any withdrawals. Instead, you sort of "reset" your tolerance level. Another way is to switch strains or to lower the dose again.

To Inhale, Ingest or Apply Topically?

The popularity of CBD has led to more option for patients to take their cannabis dosage. While THC has been singled out as medicinal, CBD is primarily seen as an herbal supplement because of the lack of impairment.

For inhalation, cannabinoids enter the bloodstream through the lungs. The results are usually instant and can last for 2-6 hours. For ingested cannabinoids, the absorption is much slower, not to mention the fact that compounds have to be able to survive stomach acid in high enough concentrations to be effective. The results are erratic and can take up to 2 hours to be seen. While they often last longer (6 hours or more) than inhalation, the issue of the quantity and lack of consistency makes it harder to determine whether this is a successful choice. Tinctures and drops, which are absorbed by the membranes in the mouth rather than swallowed, work quickest - in as little as 15 minutes. The problem is that the dose is also quite low and usually only lasts for around 4 hours.

Topical compounds are difficult to dose and judge by effectiveness, partially because transdermal options are usually made of higher grade medical CBD. Because most topical applications don't reach the bloodstream, the effectiveness is only localized. Transdermal medications often last longer, with 12 hours reported, though the effectiveness diminishes over time.

Because taking CBD is very individualized, the standards and potency often fluctuate wildly. With each strain, application, and product being almost as unique as the patient, dosage can be difficult if you're looking for specific benefits compared to THC.

The closer we get to legalization, the more these methods of delivery can be refined and even enlarged to suit users. The array of options is daunting for most first-time users, and the only way you can make a choice is by understanding your options and determining the best CBD dosing method for yourself before trying it. To be safest, using your intuition and the principal of starting small before building up, you can record how your body reacts and adjust until you reach a dosage that works for you.

Tinctures

Tinctures are one of the oldest forms of "medicine". The whole plant is soaked into a carrier and brewed, often for extended periods, until the useful compounds infuse into the carrier. Carriers can be oil- or alcohol-based, but they are always liquid by nature. A standard tincture dose usually comes in a 0.5oz-2oz container. A dropper or small syringe makes it easier to be accurate with dosing. For alcohol-based tinctures, 25-30 drops is the average therapeutic dose, with a product that is 10-20 mg/ml in strength, but since tinctures can be as high as 50 mg/ml for CBD, it's important not to jump into the high 30 drop dose immediately.

Taking tinctures is usually done orally, either as a spray into the throat, drops under the tongue, in capsules, or added to food. It is very strong-tasting, with a bitter and particularly unpleasant flavor.

The alcohol used is also usually 190-proof, which means strong and burning. Many people don't like using tinctures because of their unpleasant taste, not to mention the fact that the concentration can be irritating to delicate mouth membranes. If you're using an alcohol-based tincture, you can also add it into a drink that has a sour taste to diffuse it such as citrus juice, tea, or even just plain water, though you may still want to rinse it to get rid of the taste. It's less common to mix it with soft or sweet food, but it can be done.

A tincture usually takes at least 30 minutes to take effect, but it lasts for 6-8 hours. Dosing is usually done 3 times a day but can be as often as six times. The ideal dose is strong enough that it can be felt but low enough to not take over the user's lucidity. Naturally, the effects are stronger on an empty stomach.

CBD is commonly found as an oil tincture because it is easily infused into the oil. It is usually done with some form of edible oil. Because the oil acts as a protective layer, this is easier to take directly into the mouth for absorption before it reaches the stomach acid. Unlike alcohol-based tinctures, oil mixtures do not mix well with juice or drinks but will mix into heavier foods like soup or yogurt. The dosage is the same, but the effects take longer to be felt. The shelf life of oils is much shorter than alcohol tinctures.

A less common type of tincture using glycerin can also be found - they are best for those who have an intolerance to alcohol.

Sublingual Spray/Strips

These are very fast-acting, with less than 2 minutes for the effects to be felt, but they last just as long as other orally used CBD products. The number of blood vessels within the mouth is high enough that a significant amount is absorbed before being swallowed, and it is one of the best ways to make the cannabinoids in CBD bioavailable. It also delivers a similar speed to that of smoking or vaporizing without having to deal with the side effects of smoking like dry mouth and smell.

Much like breath strips, sublingual strips are equally fast-acting and dissolve within a couple of minutes. Like with the spray, the effects usually last 6-8 hours and are more bioavailable because they bypass the liver and digestive system. Each strip comes in a measured dose and may be flavored between 5-40mg of CBD per strip.

Capsules

Capsules are often tinctures and powders which are concentrated and then packaged into a small capsule shell. This gives a premeasured dose and is much more accurate compared to tinctures and sublinguals. Capsules take up to 90 minutes to take effect and can be effective for up to 8 hours. They are better for long-term use because they provide a much more consistent level of CBD. While most people have no issues with capsules, there is a small percentage of users who have issues with the raw plant materials used.

Edibles

The iconic "pot brownie" is a rather fun way to take your medicine. It's one of the fastest growing areas of research because we all love to eat but hate taking medicine, so doing both together makes a much more enjoyable experience. Edibles come in numerous shapes and sizes and are usually sweet rather than savory. Edibles are usually made with raw plant or oil infusions.

The downside of many edibles is that they're often made using cannabis that has been extracted with alcohol or CO2. This means it's less pure than the tincture or capsule form and incredibly hard to dose accurately. It can take several hours before effects are felt, and this also means that often people are tempted to take more, thinking that the edibles aren't working. While taking too much CBD isn't going to cause adverse effects, it can be uncomfortable and dosing can last longer than necessary.

Another downside to edibles is that they are often attractive to pets and children. We've all heard of the Halloween candy warning!

Lozenges

Much like a combination of capsules and tinctures, lozenges are not meant to be swallowed but kept in the mouth until they dissolve. They take about 20 minutes to take effect and dissolve fully within several minutes, which adds to their effectiveness. CBD lozenges have between 10-20mg of CBD per dose and are usually honey-based to disguise the taste. They're much like cough medicine and may have soothing herbs like Echinacea added.

Concentrated Oil

This is the most recognized form of CBD treatments, coming in a small essential oil bottle or a measured syringe. It can be mixed with other oils to make a carrier and then made into edibles or capsules. The benefit of the concentrated oil is that for patients who need a stronger dose, this is the only way to get that effect. Each concentrated oil is between 50-75% CBD, with a single drop containing up to 50mg of CBD. The oil is usually quite thick and dark. The syringe allows for easier application than the oil bottle and often has measurement lines. It's impossible to get a small dose using the concentrated oil so this should only be used by patients looking for this high a dosage.

Raw Cannabis Juice

The juicing craze has also reached CBD. It's much less likely you'll find CBD in this form because it's usually a whole plant approach. Raw cannabis juice is untreated, which means it also contains the acids CBDA and THCA, the precursors to CBD and THC. Because these acids are non-psychoactive it's possible to eat them and not get “high” despite ingesting a THC compound. These have been shown to have similar properties to THC and CBD but because the whole plant is being used, you're also getting the effects of a variety of other compounds within the plant. Cannabis juice should be consumed within 12 hours and while it can be frozen, the crystallization process can damage the molecules.

Smoking

The most recognized form of taking medical marijuana nowadays is smoking. Inhaling cannabinoids has an instant effect. When choosing plants for CBD therapy, it's important to get the right strains, like Cannatonic, Remedy, Valentine X, Charlotte's Web, Harlequin, or Sour Tsunami.

The most common methods of smoking are cigarettes or joints. These are traditionally rolled using thin paper, and it's the fastest method for the body to absorb CBD. The problem is smokers have to deal with the intense taste and the strong odor that tends to linger. However, there is no research that has successfully linked smoking marijuana to lung cancer despite of what early propaganda said.

Cannabis pipes are also fairly common and come in a variety of different and even makeshift shapes. Small pipes are made for single, lower dose use because the amount of cannabis that can be used at any time is small. A water pipe is one of the most common types and has been around for about 2,400 years. It works by passing the smoke through water before inhaling it, which acts as a filter for toxins and potential impurities. Using a water pipe is less irritating because the smoke is cooler, but it also requires the apparatus to be cleaned and maintained and the water to be changed regularly.

Vaporizing or "Vaping"

Like smoking, vaporizing heats the cannabis to release cannabinoids without the harmful effects and byproducts that smoking may have. Vaping is often preferred to smoking, partially because of the popularity of the method and because vapor usually lacks the traditional smell of marijuana, allowing it to be combined with other masking scents for a more discreet use. CBD boils at a higher temperature than THC, which means it can maintain a greater flavor profile than smoking.

A vaporizer usually has one of two heating elements - conduction or convection, much like a kitchen oven. Small vape pens and portable vaporizers are usually conduction-heated for convenience and size. These are direct-draw, which means a user can simply inhale the smoke by using the mouthpiece over the heating element.

There are no known adverse health effects to vape pens, but depending on your inhalation style, you may take a stronger dose than expected, depending on the oil. The known issue with vaping is that one of the additives in CBD oil cartridges, propylene glycol, has been linked to becoming formaldehyde (a carcinogen) when heated and inhaled. This means that while the heated CBD vape oil itself isn't harmful, the additive may be.

Topical Lotions/Salves

Topical or transdermal cannabis is often used for localized pain, muscle soreness and arthritis. This is a non-psychoactive form and the least invasive, but it is only effective for complaints that are within 1″ of the skin depth since they can't reach further. Extreme conditions like skin cancer require higher doses than most topical solutions provide.

Transdermal patches are the exception - they have a high enough concentration to permeate the skin and reach the blood stream. The effect of topical medicines lasts 6-8 hours.

Suppositories

This is one of the more unusual dosing methods, and while it's been used for centuries it is best for conditions of the colon and lower bowel, where a stomach dosage may not survive long enough to reach. This provides a bioavailable medication through rectal or vaginal tissue and is most useful for patients who have cancers of the lower abdomen like rectal, prostate, colon, or ovarian cancer. It's also a fairly large dose application since it's usually made using concentrated oil mixed with cocoa butter, and it can last 7 hours or more.

Young Patients

Unlike THC, CBD is often used for patients under 22 because there is less chance of developing a dependence on it and affecting IQ or academic performance. Heavy usage of THC products at a young age has been shown to do both, though tobacco usage is still a greater risk. Most companies refuse to allow patients under 18 to receive CBD or cannabis products because the brain is still developing at that age.

Chapter 5 – CBD and Healing the Brain

Despite not having any psychoactive effects, CBD does have distinct links to affecting the brain. Many people use it to treat anxiety, PTSD, attention disorders and to regulate their moods.

CBD for Anxiety

We have all experienced stress at some point. Many people use marijuana because it makes them feel less stressed and mellower. The issue is that marijuana often has the side effect of causing paranoia, which doesn't help if you're already anxious. The reason CBD is superior is that it is the active component that works against the paranoia-inducing THC in medical marijuana.

Anxiety can mean a range of different disorders but in the most severe cases, it means that the person is debilitated by the stress within their brain. This can either be real stress or imagined, but their response to it is heightened well above normal levels. Most conventional medications have nasty side effects or are highly addictive. The issue with conventional medication is that, like cannabidiol, each person's receptors are unique, so there's still no one treatment for anxiety. The link between the paranoia of marijuana and lowered anxiety is thought to be because of the way endocannabinoids work. The level of endocannabinoids in the blood has shown that people who have lots of CB1 receptors are also very susceptible to levels of the chemical GABA. GABA is a neurotransmitter which regulates stress vs reward when it comes to experience. Endocannabinoids regulate the level of GABA and other hormones and act as a buffer to extreme highs or lows. In a normal stress response, anxiety is temporarily heightening and part of the "fight or flight" response to danger or fear. It's thought that anxiety is an incorrect or prolonged perception of danger (where none actually exists) within the body. When the stress response is permanently high, the body can't keep producing endocannabinoids or becomes desensitized to them (research isn't sure yet). Ingesting

cannabinoids boosts the available chemicals to interact with those receptors and thereby lowers the GABA response.
This is also the reason why CBD is commonly linked with PTSD. By stifling the "danger" response, PTSD patients are less likely to re-experience the stress of their trauma because the brain isn't being triggered to produce the same fight or flight response that has become normal. Studies on CBD showed that patients who were given CBD versus conventional anxiety medications had the same blood flow patterns and same feelings regardless of their "treatment".

CBD for Depression

Depression, like anxiety, is not wholly understood. Depression can usually be attributed to a chemical imbalance within the brain or the chemicals it produces. The main chemicals linked to mood are serotonin and dopamine, levels of which regulate our ability to stay "happy", motivation, and a host of other processes. Conventional depression medications focusses on serotonin and dopamine with the most common being SSRIs and SSIs - Selective Serotonin Reuptake Inhibitors and Serotonin Reuptake Inhibitors, which stop the body from using up as much of the serotonin in the blood.

Serotonin is a neurotransmitter. It is responsible for helping the brain pass messages from one nerve to the next and making those messages pass more frequently so that the message is complete and understood by the next cell. Research has tentatively linked CBD with boosting the number of transmissions within the brain. Aside from the fact that most depression medications have terrible side effects, CBD has also been shown to have a faster effect on serotonin levels and greater compatibility with the 5-HT1A receptors that SSIs and SSRIs interact with.

The reason CBD is used to treat depression is that it covers a wide range of symptoms that people experience with depression, such as loss of appetite, lack of motivation, bad mood, physical pain, and anxiety. CBD has proven effective against all these.

Addiction

Addiction is often referred to as a brain disease because many people with mental health issues also struggle with addiction. Cannabis is often dubbed addictive, but there is little evidence to support this claim, especially if compared to narcotics. High THC strains, however, have led to some patients developing mental dependence. The potential for abuse exists because of this. These same strains can also cause withdrawal symptoms. CBD doesn't have these risks and can actually be used to treat nicotine, alcohol, and other drug addictions by helping soothe the anxiety caused by withdrawal and to help ease the mental anguish that may have led to the addicting behavior in the first place.

Chapter 6 – CBD & Pain

Everyone knows what pain is. Some people are unlucky enough that they live their lives in constant pain. Our brains are designed not only to process pain but to make the experience less traumatic. When we are in pain, our bodies release a host of chemicals, including endocannabinoids, to lessen what we feel, and then our body is programmed to simply forget. While we can remember the experience of being in pain, it's physically impossible to re-experience the actual physical sensation we underwent once before. However, for those with chronic pain, the pain never goes away.

Pain comes from a variety of sources, which is why CBD isn't always effective. It's thought that the reason it sometimes works with little "reason" is in the number of CBD receptors a patient has. For patients with higher CB2 receptors, if their naturally produced endocannabinoids are not high enough to counteract the pain the body simply can't do anything about, it adds cannabinoids to boost this number so that the body has enough to lessen the pain.

How Pain Works

There are 5 types of pain recognized by doctors - acute pain, chronic pain, nociceptive pain, neuropathic pain and psychogenic pain. Each type is triggered by different things, and not all of them are physical. Within each type of pain, the level experienced is also divided into classifications of severity.

Acute pain is sudden and limited and often caused by damaging the body in some way -like a broken bone for instance. It causes emotional distress and is similar to nociceptive pain. The difference it that acute pain is much more severe and debilitating. You've probably seen someone suddenly double over in pain because of a wrong movement - that's acute pain. It's not the same as being punched in the face, where the pain will pass again in due time.

Chronic pain can be either sharp or dull, but instead of it going away it stays for long periods of time. It may also be resistant to common treatments and in the case of some diseases, the reason for the pain itself isn't apparent. Chronic pain is usually the result of nerve damage and can severely affect a person's mind. Depression and anxiety are both linked to chronic pain as well as flare-ups, where the pain breaks through even when medication is used.

Nociceptive pain is intense pain usually caused by an injury. It becomes worse when the damaged area is moved and is specific to tissue damage rather than nerve damage. Tissue damage is a vague classification as conditions like cancer can also be classified as tissue damage. It can feel like an ache or throbbing in minor cases.

Neuropathic pain is mainly caused by damaged nerves. Sciatica, for example, is one of the most commonly recognizable nerve pains. The nerve may simply be trapped or pinched, but it's triggering a sharp, lightning-like pain response. Nerves act much like power cables so when there is damage, the cable "sparks" send incomplete or abnormal messages. Nerves can be damaged by chemotherapy drugs, trauma, infections, or a brain injury, which controls everything that can send faulty pain messages. Nerve pain is usually a burning or prickling sensation with occasional spikes of sharp pain. Patients also may have hypersensitivity to touch.

Psychogenic pain often goes hand in hand with depression. While there is no physical cause for psychogenic pain, it can still have physical symptoms. It can arise from fear, stress, depression, or anxiety but has an entirely psychological basis.

Why the Type of Pain Is Important for CBD

CBD is a common treatment for pain, but it can't treat all pain. Saying CBD treats pain is like saying that antibiotics kill infection - it's technically true, but there's specifics involved. CBD can treat pain in a variety of ways - by increasing the cannabinoids so that your body doesn't feel the pain so strongly anymore, by settling mental anguish, by improving nerve transmission, and by improving your mood so that the "forgetting" process can kick in.
Understanding how pain works at its most basic level holds the key to why CBD is effective.

Pain is felt through the nerves when they are activated or triggered. The trigger sends a message up through the nerve and spine and into the brain. The receptor for pain is then triggered using neurotransmitter chemicals, and the message is interpreted by the brain as a physical and mental experience. Ouch! This all happens in a split second, which is why you can often remove yourself from whatever is causing the pain before you even feel it. You've probably jerked your hand away from a hot pot before without having experienced an actual burn. This happens when the message reaches your muscles faster than your thoughts - that's when your survival instinct kicks in.

The reason CBD will not work on all the types of pain is that when the pain is not caused by an interruption of these messages, incorrect messages, or mental distress affecting the messages, there is nothing CBD can do. For example, if you break a bone, CBD can make the messages travel to your brain to better interpret the pain, but you'll still feel it because the nerves and tissue are damaged. It isn't like an opioid painkiller because it doesn't block the pain messages from making it to the brain so you'll still feel it.

Chronic pain is the perfect candidate for CBD treatment because it is usually related to nerve transmission. The same is true of neuropathic and psychogenic pain because they all relate to the nerves and how pain messages are relayed through the body.

CBD as an Analgesic

CBD doesn't just work on neurotransmitters by mimicking essential chemicals. It can also act to lower inflammation. Inflammation of the neural pathways is considered to be one of the reasons for chronic pain and neuropathic pain. When pain receptors become inflamed, either through disease or damage, they are triggered so it makes sense that lowering or targeting that inflammation lessens the body's pain response.

Long-term use of anti-inflammatory drugs has been linked to severe side effects, which is why many people are hesitant to use them. However, the modern lifestyle is full of inflammatory foods and chemicals so they're pretty much impossible to avoid.

As an analgesic, CBD isn't reducing pain. It's reducing the inflammation that causes a pain response. This is why it's only effective for limited types of pain. THC is actually much more effective as an anti-inflammatory; in fact, about 20 times more effective than aspirin. The main anti-inflammatory in CBD is cannabichromene, and it's not as strong or effective as similar compounds in THC. This is where medical marijuana has an edge compared to CBD because it is more effective at reducing inflammation.

Cannabis contains β-sitosterol, a phytosterol which has anti-inflammatory properties. B-sitosterol has also been shown to have strong links with skin cells and improving the condition of the skin. Since most pain receptors are located close to the skin, this could also be the reason that CBD is so effective for nerve pain and, more specifically, diseases like fibromyalgia.

Cancer

Many people have touted cannabis as a "cure" for cancer, and dying people will believe anything if they think it might save them. It's cruel, but **there is no known cure for cancer** yet. However, studies have shown links to reversing the damage from cancer, which is why it's been called curative. Many other things that date as far back as 1904 have successfully "cured" cancer by killing cancer cells. In theory, you can "cure" cancer cells by pouring bleach on them but it wouldn't be very healthy for the patient.

There are hundreds of different types of cancer and thousands of different causes. Treating cancer is frustrating for medical professionals because even the most promising treatments aren't always effective.

The widely accepted reason of how cancer works is that cells mutate during their life cycle. This mutation causes abnormal cells that would normally be destroyed but instead multiply and spread, causing other wrong cells to disrupt the body's natural processes.

Aside from treating the chronic pain associated with cancer, CBD studies have shown that the oil has a similar effect on shrinking tumors to that of chemotherapy but without the nasty side effects. The same studies showed a similar effect to opioids for treating the pain.

Dr. Donald Adams, a noted oncologist who supports CBD therapy, also admits that it's not a cure. If patients administered CBD oil had a significantly higher rate of survival than those who weren't, then it could be considered a cure, but that isn't the case since statistics have remained the same. That doesn't mean that CBD can't improve their life though.

Even medical marijuana can't cure cancer, though the effects are similar to those of CBD on cancer patients. For those studies that have "cured" cancer, it's often a case of having ideal conditions. Since most cancer tests are done in a lab rather than on human subjects, the results are under "optimum" conditions, which would be almost impossible to replicate in the body, especially when someone isn't in "optimum" health.

As far as science goes, CBD is considered therapeutic but not curative despite having anti-cancer properties. Studies have shown that THC actually causes certain cancer cells to implode, while cannabinoid compounds block cell growth and prevent tumors from spreading. Especially for prostate cancer cells, which are independent of testosterone and more prone to spreading, CBD is better as a treatment because it doesn't just cause the implosion but creates a whole approach therapy that stops from cancer progressing and metastasizing.

Chapter 7 – CBD Recipes & Life

It's important when you're considering taking any form of cannabis to know how much. While there's never been such a thing as a marijuana overdose, overuse can cause long-term damage to the body. Most physicians are hesitant to suggest or prescribe cannabis treatments because there isn't an "official" dosage and medical schools certainly haven't covered that in pharmacology. Science is only now starting to create a dosing schedule and amount that makes any sense and even with this information without knowing the number of CB receptors in your own body the dose may not be ideal.

Recommended Dose

Another reason the recommended dose is difficult to figure out is that many brands have completely different suggestions. The recommended "serving" of CBD oil differs from brand to brand, just like the amount of THC in marijuana strains can differ.

With dried cannabis, it's almost impossible to determine the exact amount of cannabinoids because doing so destroys the product and since the amount can differ from plant to plant and strain to strain, proper dosing is a dilemma.
CBD usually comes in drop or tincture form. The drop or extract oil is much more potent than the tincture, but you should look on your product information for the mg of cannabinoids and go by that rather than a specific X drops per day amount. If your body isn't getting the benefits, adjust that amount accordingly so that *you* feel its effects. Do not simply assume that each brand has the same amount of cannabinoids just because the bottles are the same size. Start with the smallest dose. Since there is a possibility of allergy and everyone's reaction will be different, a negative reaction at this level indicates that it's probably not safe to use a higher dose or any at all.
A general dosing guide for CBD:

- General Health Use : ~2.5-15mg/day
- Chronic Pain Use: ~2.5-20mg/day
- Sleep and Anxiety Use: ~40-160mg/day

Remember, these are not necessarily accurate or appropriate for *you*, and you should always build towards a high dose to prevent side effects.

Topical Cannabinoids

Our skin is a porous membrane, and many things can pass through it to treat disease or damage beneath. Cannabinoids are so tiny that they can go through the pores, meaning using CBD or cannabis treatments topically may be even more effective than drops or smoke inhalation. CBD tends to be the preferred cannabinoid source for topical use as it's just as fast and doesn't have the psychoactive effects, but many recipes can be made with dried cannabis instead.

When doing crafts or cooking with CBD, the infused oil is actually the best kind. It's much like adding coconut oil or cocoa butter to a recipe rather than pure cannabinoids and will sustain any heating process better than the tincture.

Do not cook anything above 350 degrees, or it will degrade the compounds. Even then, cook 10-15 degrees below that to include temperature fluctuations. The first recipe uses oil infused with CBD directly from buds, which is only legal in states with medical marijuana laws. A typical dose of THC is 10mg, so having a higher dose will likely give you more of the THC than the CBD effects, regardless of what strain you use.

CBD Salve

Ingredients:

1oz beeswax
1oz refined shea or coconut butter
1cup canna oil

Using a double boiler, add the oil and get the water to simmer. Break in beeswax and stir until almost completely dissolved, then add coconut or shea butter. Break into small pieces so it melts quicker. You can also add a few drops of essential oil for scent as it will smell like cannabis otherwise - herbal scents like rosemary and lavender work well. Pour the oil mixture into liquid- and heat-proof containers like tins or glass jars and allow to sit until solid. Do not freeze or refrigerate. Store in a cool location and use within 6 months.

CBD Cookies

Ingredients:

8oz baking cocoa or dark chocolate
1stick unsalted butter
1c milk
2/3c all-purpose flour
1/2tsp baking powder
Pinch of salt
2 Eggs
1/2c packed light brown sugar

1/2c sugar
1tsp vanilla extract
1tsp CBD oil
12oz chocolate chips

Preheat the oven to 300°F. Beat eggs and sugar until smooth; add CBD and vanilla and mix well; then set aside. In a double boiler, melt butter and add milk. Stir well, then add cocoa and continue to stir until it has melted and blended. Remove from heat and combine with eggs until fully mixed, then mix in dry ingredients and chocolate chips. Roll into 24 balls and place on a cookie sheet with parchment paper. Bake 18-20 minutes, then remove and allow to cool. Store in an airtight container for up to 1 week.

CBD for Dietary Issues

While making and using edibles is one of the most common methods of CBD dosing, it is often used to help with dietary problems because of the direct application to the digestive system. Several studies have shown that those who use cannabis products have a lower BMI and a lower risk for obesity and diabetes. A 2011 study determined that only 1/3 of users were at risk for obesity despite the population at large being at a 1 in 2 risk. Despite the common "joke" about cannabis and "munchies", CBD doesn't usually stimulate the appetite enough to consume excessively because it is usually the THC's stimulant effect that does this.

CBD on its own has been shown to aid diabetics by helping the body convert white fat into brown fat, which regulates insulin levels better and helps with metabolism. Most cannabis users have a fasting insulin level that is significantly lower than those who do not use and were found to be more sensitive to insulin changes. Even those who had already given up cannabis had the same advantage, though it became less pronounced over time, something that may show a protective effect instead.

Because of the anti-inflammatory properties of CBD, it can also be used to treat IBS and Crohn's since these diseases are primarily triggered by foods causing inflammation in the gut.

CBD for Pets

Many low dose CBD products are also suitable for pets. Elderly dogs and those with cancer are most often used as study patients, and the effects are much the same as those in their human counterparts. However, it's no surprise that few veterinarians are willing to back treatments just yet.

The dosing schedules discussed earlier in the book using titration can be just as effective for pets. Your primary goal should be determining which products are safest and most effective for your pet based on ratio and concentration. A high CBD dose is best for serious conditions such as cancer, seizures, and various types of pain.

With the expectation that cannabis medications will become more widely available in the near future, it seems inevitable that there will be some for pets too, but a complete overhaul of the law probably won't happen for quite some time.

Conclusion

Thank you for buying this book. I've tried to include information that I felt was missing from other books and back it up with real science to convince skeptics of CBD success. Even if you've decided CBD oil isn't for you, you can hopefully at least accept that it works well for others.

It's true that CBD isn't for everyone, and the fact that it's not legal everywhere yet is a problem. It's important to know the difference between THC and CBD as they are not the same thing, just like hemp and cannabis are not exactly the same.

CBD is not a cure; it cannot make diseases go away, but it can ease your symptoms and your pain without many of the nasty side effects that conventional medicine entails.

If you enjoyed my book or learned something from it, go ahead and leave a review. It will be much appreciated. I know CBD isn't for everyone, and until marijuana is legal for medical purposes in all states, it's still a "drug" for many people.

I hope my book has helped you as much as it helped me, and one day we may be lucky enough that everyone can enjoy the benefits of cannabis.

-Allan

Thank again for your support through buying and reading this book, it means the world to me!

If you never want to miss out on one of my future books, consider signing up for my newsletter here

http://bit.ly/allannewsletter

and checking out my author's page here

http://amzn.to/allanmccampbell

Made in the USA
Middletown, DE
08 October 2018